Meditation for Beginners

The Complete Guide to Meditation Benefits on Health and How to Meditate for Beginners

By Kristy McMillan

Contents

This book *"**Meditation for Beginners**",* is written to educate you on the importance and benefits of *Meditation with Practical Tips & Practice That Enhances Mindfulness and Sense of Calm hence Good Health*, get your energy back, boost your productivity, and get focused in general.

I really had no idea what meditation was or even how to get started. A few years ago everything was crumbling around me. I lost my mom and left some other relationships I felt were toxic to me and some old symptoms of PTSD started to pop up (I was assaulted as a child , stabbed in the chest actually) I also have a chronic illness, which has the potential to become worse and require a certain type of brain surgery, and even then there is no guarantee it will be fixed. The stress level was sky high. Something kept drawing me to meditation. But what was it? It looks like it's just doing nothing. To just sit down, close your eyes, and do nothing. Sorry, that's just not how this mind of mine works! I was the type of person who would find something to analyze but still, something kept drawing me to it so I felt the need to at least try. So is it sitting and doing nothing? Sort of. There is a little more to it. You can massively improve your life, and more importantly, the way you feel about your life by meditating. And for the most part, it does just involve sitting down and doing nothing, so how does it work? How can it have such profound effect on us? Is it easy?

Meditation can be a difficult or should I say an uncomfortable habit to build, especially if you've never done it before. Like I stated above, my mind was always on the go. I literally had no idea what it was like to not be analyzing SOMEthing. Now that I have the hang of it I felt the need to share. This is to help you start meditating, even if you've never done it before. I just want you to get the feeling, to have some idea of what it is. I am also a nurse so I am going to throw in some of the health benefits as well!

Introduction

Meditation is a practice that is used to achieve greater mastery of the mind, so that it becomes able to focus on a single thought, on a high concept, or a precise element of reality, ceasing its usual chattering of the background and becoming absolutely quiet and peaceful. Similar to meditation is contemplation, which is the ability to let the mind rest in its natural state. Therefore, it is a practice aimed at self-realization, which can have religious, spiritual or philosophical impact. In reflective meditation the object of meditation can be anything. Generally speaking, during practice the visualization of elements that concern the inner world or simple objects are used, to reach a greater state of concentration and grounding. This type of meditation is very popular in the Western culture.

On the other hand, receptive meditation aims at the absence of thoughts and allows the mind to reach a level of "mindless awareness", that is free from the psychic activity of the human being, which can be chaotic and confusing. It is more used in the Eastern culture and a little harder to tap in to, in my opinion. There are many personal paths that do not come from a specific religion or a philosophy and of which meditation is a fundamental tool to deepen and develop the hidden side of ourselves. It is a great way to 'receive." Just WHAT you may receive really depends on your personal belief system, but I digress.

A fundamental aspect in meditation is the reduction of suffering. This is extremely relevant to us, as every technique described in the next chapters aim at entering a deeper state of mind, where suffering is not excluded, but managed and controlled from a quieter place. There will always be suffering, especially in the current world we live in. There is no amount of meditation (that I am aware of) that can put an end to that, but I am satisfied that I am doing my part to not take on every burden in the world. I have learned what is mine to carry and what is NOT mine to carry. Only those who do not know how to master their feelings and emotions, try to avoid suffering; the ones that know themselves, find immense opportunity in it. I will say that I used to be the former, but there are some things that are out of one's control and when you are forced to join the latter, you will seek and seek until you find something to bring you peace.

Chapter 1: Why Practice Meditation?

Well, after reading all that, don't you want to practice it just to see how it works and to get those benefits? I will explain a bit more about it here. Meditation bestows a host of benefits on its practitioner from the very start. Some are fairly obvious, like increased awareness of one's own mind and body. Others are often touted but sometimes not clearly explained, like relief from anxiety, depression, panic attacks and other mental illnesses. Perhaps this is due to a hesitance to accept non-western medicinal approaches to these things, though they are growing in popularity as healing skills, with both the medical community and the world at large. Like I stated before, I am a Registered Nurse in the Western medicine system, but there came a time in my life where all of the medications just were not cutting it. Most of the side effects led to more issues. And when I read that meditation can also increase your energy and focus, help you change your behaviors, and improve your quality of work and exercise I said "Sign Me Up!!"It can even improve your immunity and overall health, let's be honest here, who couldn't stand to have that happen ?

What Effect Does It Have on Your Brain?

Not only does meditation help you focus on the right stuff, but it makes your thought patterns faster, stronger, and more in your control. The 'fight or flight' response is the reaction most of us have to a stressful situation. In the past it was very useful, for example if we see a tiger, we don't have time to think about it, we just need to run. And in the past, this fight or flight response was critical for keeping us alive. But today? Well, there aren't many tigers roaming the streets, and the world's a lot safer in that respect.. Most of us don't experience danger every day. However, most of us sadly use the same fight or flight response when we experience petty, pointless stress like road rage or arriving late to work. We've somehow managed to evolve to the point where we get stressed on an emotional and physical level, by things that really don't matter and don't affect our chances of survival at all. Things that really shouldn't have any effect on our emotional state and certainly not on our physical bodies and systems.

Remember, the fight or flight response has its place. If you're in a street fight or there's a natural disaster, yes you need that response. You need to be able to react, and move fast in order to protect yourself from harm. And it will be there for you when you need it. But most of us are reacting to an angry boss at work in the same way physically that we'd react to a vicious bear attacking us! The same hormones, stress responses, chemicals and processes are happening in our bodies in this situation! This means our bodies are experiencing more stress than ever before, because we've lost touch with our ability to be in our bodies and not our minds. By being so focused on our minds, and our thoughts, we've lost the ability to be in our bodies. If we were in our bodies, your angry boss wouldn't matter at all. You'd probably laugh at how angry they're getting; I know I sometimes do! It's almost silly how angry people get at seemingly pointless or insignificant things.

When you experience the fight or flight response, your body pumps hormones like adrenaline and epinephrine through your veins. Your lungs expand and take in more oxygen and if you perceive the stress is still be there after a few seconds, you get even more. It's like a gas pedal being held down while the car isn't moving. After a while it burns the engine out, so now imagine the effect of that gas pedal being held down in your body for years on end. It's not good, I can tell you that. It's actually very bad for your body and mind and over time, it can make you sick. And it does! Chronic stress, which is stress experience in little amounts over a long period of time can make your immune system weaker. Think about this the next time you're angry at someone cutting in front of you in traffic. By getting angry, you're literally making yourself ill. Just flip them off and let it go! I am kidding there (or am I?)

It's quite funny to think about this. We're one of the most intelligent species (apparently) on the planet, and we for some reason choose to make ourselves ill and stressed because someone cut in front of us in traffic for a split second. It's crazy. We've become blind to what we're doing. Or, we'll get angry if the waiter brings us the wrong food by accident. This is how we actually behave in the world today! We choose to experience this stress, and it IS a choice. When you learn about meditation, and once you've read this book, you'll have the choice of how to react to situations like that. The fight or flight response interestingly, uses that same 'default mode network' It involves the amygdala, and produces hormones that flood your body with rage, energy and so on. It's useful for an actual fight or a situation in which you need to sprint to get away from danger. But it's pointless, and actually harmful to have that same response when your boss shouts at you, you're late for work, or the waiter brings you chips instead of soup.

So, if the fight of flight response is not needed for 99% of our lives, how can we keep those stress hormones from pumping through our body and wreaking havoc? It's very harmful. So, specifically, mindfulness meditation can actually shrink the part of your brain responsible for 'fight or flight' responses, which tend to be more emotional and not thought through. While it also strengthens your higher brain functions which happen in the frontal pre-cortex. This means you're more able to think on a higher level about things logically and reasonably. This means our normal responses to stress that we can't seem to control, are completely different. We're able, after just 8 weeks of meditation, to have much greater control over our thoughts and emotions in times of stress. Listen, this really works. I feel I have really been able to balance myself out by meditating and practicing mindfulness.

Let's get back to the results of stress on the body. The brain notices the oncoming onslaught of perceived annoyance before I've really realized what's happening consciously. A distress signal gets sent to my amygdala (in the default mode network, remember?). The amygdala works out that I'm in danger, and instantly sends a distress signal to my hypothalamus. That area of the brain is sort of like a command or control room. It decides how to act and it does all of this in tiny fractions of a second. It's incredible. This means the hormones remain in the system, and they stay amped up with high blood pressure and so on. Maybe you've experienced a situation where you're so annoyed, angry and stressed that you just can't sit still. You feel it flowing through your veins, right?

That's the hormones your brain is telling your body to give you, because it thinks you're in danger! It says "OH MY GOD WHY is this person in front of me driving 35 mph when the speed limit is 35 mph!! I am going to be late!" It says " I can't believe this waiter brought me my water with ABSOLUTELY no lemon!" Now obviously, I am exaggerating a wee bit and I do know that there are times when there are actual things to stress over but my point is your body thinks you're about to have a fight or run for your life and it's supplying you with these hormones to give you energy. But if you don't use them or need them, the effect they have on your body is very harmful. Anyway, meditation helps you reduce that, so that you only get those stress hormones when you really need them to save your life. You won't catch me getting worked up over a meal that's late, or somebody cutting me off in traffic. It just won't happen because I value my health and mental and emotional state way more than that.

One thing I found extremely interesting about meditation is that it can actually help you experience less pain. I want to share with you that I have a medical condition called trigeminal neuralgia. You can google it to see exactly what it is and what it does but it really says something when its nickname is "the Suicide Disease". I was diagnosed about 6 years ago and have suffered immensely. I can safely say that I lived in chronic pain nearly every day. There is no rhyme or reason to this condition and I cannot control when the flare ups happen. Meditation has really helped me to cope with this and actually, the last time I saw my neurologist she was amazed that I had not had my narcotic pain medications filled in over a year and I shared with her how meditation was actually helping me to not really need them as often. How? In the brains of advanced meditators, the pain centers of the brain actually light up more, but the people report feeling less pain. How can that be? It's a paradox, but it seems that meditation somehow helps people experience less pain. It does this in a very complex way. The way it works, is that mediators have actually decoupled (weakened) the link between the anterior cingulate cortex (area of the brain responsible for unpleasantness of pain) and the prefrontal cortex. That means they still feel the pain but it's much less. The effect of pain in most people, in largely in the mind. There is some nervous system pain which is unavoidable, but the rest of the 'pain experience' we've all come to know is made up in the brain. It's a response to the real pain, and it can make it up to 10 times worse.

In a lot of people, there is a loop which means you constantly re-experience the same pain. But in meditators, this loop is mainly closed down. They're still aware of the pain, but it's much less than non-meditators. Amazingly, this effect can be seen even when people aren't meditating, meaning the meditation has caused a permanent change in their brain and the way they experience pain. This also applies to the lowered stress response. It seems meditation can physically change the brain for the better in just a few weeks. Now imagine having meditated for decades. It's no wonder that Buddhist monks are able to focus for days on end, seemingly be immune to pain, and even have control over their entire immune system and the intricate processes in their bodies. I don't know if you've seen the videos of the devoted Buddhist monks able to channel pain and strength around their bodies. One such video showed a monk resisting a sharpened spear to the throat simply by the power of intention and meditation. Now that's taken years to get to that point, but not everyone can get there. Frankly, I don't think I need to go that far but it would be a pretty cool story to tell the grandkids!

As described before, there are so many ways in which meditation improves mental health. It can assist in treating mental illnesses like depression and generalized anxiety disorder. Additionally, it can ease the chronic stress and distractibility most modern people struggle to master. Focus at work increases, and relationships with others improve. It allows you to build better connections and really listen and care what someone's saying. In short, meditation allows one to be relaxed, present, patient, and grow in wisdom and faith. Mindlessness, stress and anxiety are shown to damage the immune system and slow the recovery of injuries. They also slow the progress of weight loss, strength training and learning. A mind at peace is a mind capable of just about anything. Working to practice mindfulness pays huge dividends. Here are just a few other things you'll experience:

Better Sleep:

Meditators are able to sleep better and relax deeper. This can lead to all sorts of interesting effects, like lucid dreams (being able to control the dreams and decide what to dream about) and decreased nightmares. I suffered from insomnia for over 20 years and relied on prescription sleep medication for as many years as well. I can tell you now that I no longer need them. Most of the time I sleep like a baby.

Improved Focus:

Of course, one of the biggest benefits of meditation is being able to focus on things for long periods of time, and at an intense level. This is massively helpful if you're trying to achieve something or anything in your life.

Increases Grey Matter:

The brains of meditators are shown to actually have more grey matter. Grey matter is like the bond that holds the brain together, and helps it fire signals and process information. The greyer matter you have, the faster and better your brain operates.

Helps You Get into Flow State:

Have you ever been writing something and you just get into the 'zone'? Or maybe you've been playing a sport of working out and you just get into that headspace that's unshakable and unstoppable. You're working faster, better, and more focused, and you don't notice the time passing? That's 'flow state' and meditation helps you get there more easily and more often.

This is actually something I want to explain a bit more about. Meditation has the ability to lengthen what are known as 'telomeres' making you resistant to all sorts of diseases like Cancer and Alzheimer's! Telomeres are like the 'protective caps' on the end of your chromosomes. But wait, what's a chromosome? A chromosome is essentially a thread of protein and DNA found in the nucleus of our cells. It's pretty important. On the ends of our chromosomes are telomeres. A telomere is like the protective plastic cap on the end of a shoe lace. It stops it fraying and going all horrible. So, telomeres stop our chromosomes getting stuck together and fraying, so to speak.

Over time though, our telomeres (protective ends of our chromosomes) get shorter. This means that sooner or later, our chromosomes are no longer protected and are not able to divide or heal themselves any more. This leads to the cell dying, mutating (cancers) or changing. And this is how aging happens, our telomeres become shorter and shorter to the point where they can't effectively protect our chromosomes any more. So, our cells start dying. This is the natural aging process, but it can be slowed down massively by meditating. Meditating actually lengthens your telomeres, meaning your chromosomes are much more protected for longer. Years longer. It's like giving your individual cells a suit of armor to protect them against the passing of time, and all you need to do for that, is to sit down and do nothing for ten minutes a day!

This also means less cells die or mutate, so you look and feel younger.
But it's not just about feeling younger though. When telomeres get too short and the DNA is left exposed, it can mutate or fuse to other things. Things that it shouldn't fuse to. They can become damaged. It gets dangerous, because it can actually cause things like Cancer and other diseases. So, there are a number of things that meditation can help you with. It can lengthen telomeres and make you more resistant to things like Cancer and aging. It does this by increasing telomerase activity, which helps lengthen the telomeres attached to your DNA. Powerful stuff. But more than all of those benefits, comes the feeling of. Feeling better! Just feeling good in everyday life, and not having to worry about the stress's life or the negative aspects of life. It makes you feel good, and for a lot of people that's the most important thing. The increased focus, better sleep and immunity come as a bonus.

Chapter 2: How Meditation Works

The Mind, Body, and Meditation

Every time you meditate, you need to start off with a comfortable sitting position without any discomfort. Make sure the body is relaxed, and the head is balanced comfortably on your shoulders. Wear comfortable clothes so that you don't have any distractions whatsoever. You are aiming at not being distracted when you start the process. When it comes to meditation, how you breathe is the factor, your mind and body need to be in tune with each other while you focus on your while focusing on your breathing. Breathing helps you to center your focus on something. Studies show that focusing on deep breathing for just a while will change the mood of a person and reduce stress.

It is wise to practice meditation daily. The aim is to make sure you have a healthy emotional life that will help you deal with daily stresses. Numerous studies have shown that when you use meditation, you will decrease stress, and you get to reprogram your brain so that you have a better capacity to manage the stress. However, this only happens when you make meditation your daily practice, and you make it consistent. Before we look at the way meditating helps the stress, let us first look at how stress affects you.

The Impact of Stress

Stress doesn't only affect the mind; it goes deeper than what you might think.
Stress refers to a natural mental and physical reaction to normal life experiences. Everyone, regardless of their age or status, experiences stress at one time or another. Stress can arise from anything, including your job (hello nurse life!) and your family life (raise your hand if you have kids!!!)
For some time, especially short-term situations, stress can be good for you. It can assist you in handling potentially serious situations that can arise. The body will respond by releasing hormones that will make you react to the situation the right way. However, for the long term, and if the stress levels stay elevated, you will have chronic stress, which will cause a variety of symptoms that will affect your health the wrong way.
Some of the symptoms of chronic stress include:
- Anxiety
- Irritability
- Headaches
- Depression
- Insomnia

Stress has an effect on various parts of your body that include:

The Central Nervous System

The CNS is in control of the ability to fight or run. This is always in response to the release of stress hormones cortisol and adrenaline. When the condition is short, you will feel the thrill when your heartbeat sends blood in areas that you need in an emergency your heart, muscles, and any other vital organs. Then the fear is gone, the gland called the hypothalamus then tells your systems to go back to the normal condition. Now, here is when the issues arise when the stressor doesn't go away, and the response continues.

When the stressor maintains the reaction of the body, you are sure that you will react in a different way, including taking alcohol or getting into addiction.

The Respiratory and CVS

When stress hormones are left for so long, they will affect the respiratory system as well as the CVS. During this time, you will breathe faster so that you can distribute blood rich in oxygen around your body. For those people that have a problem with emphysema or asthma, high levels of stress make it harder for them to breath. The blood vessels will constrict so that they send more oxygen to the muscles so that you get the strength to react. The bad thing is that this also boosts your blood pressure. If the stress is prolonged, your heart will work hard and for a longer period of time. When blood pressure goes high, so does the risk of having a heart attack or a stroke.

The Digestive System

Your digestive system is also affected by stress. When under prolonged stress, the body goes ahead to produce more blood sugar that will boost your energy. However, chronic stress will make it impossible for your body to handle the regular sugar production in the body, which will, in turn, put you at risk of type 2 diabetes.

The rapid breathing, sudden rush of hormones, and the increase in the heart rate will affect the digestive system. You will experience frequent bursts of acid reflux or heartburn, a result of an increase in acid in your stomach. Stress can also affect the way food moves through the gut, which leads to constipation and diarrhea. You can also experience vomiting, nausea, or stomach pains.

The Muscular System

When you are under stress, your muscles will tense so that they protect you against injury when you get stressed. They do this voluntarily and will release when you relax, and the stress factor goes away. When your muscles are tense, you will experience body aches, headaches, shoulder, and back pain. With time, this will set off a cycle that will make you feel pain time and again.

Sexuality

Stress will exhaust you to the hilt. When you are under constant stress, you lose the desire to make love with your partner. When it is short term, men tend to produce more testosterone, but this effect doesn't last. If the stressor is prolonged, then the effects will be seen with falling testosterone levels. This can interfere with sexual prowess and can lead to impotence or erectile dysfunction. Chronic stress might also make it easy for you to develop infections. For many women, stress can lead to a change in the menstrual cycle. It can also amplify the symptoms of menopause.

The Immune System

Stress will stimulate your immune system in more ways than one. When it is an immediate situation, it can be a bonus. This stimulation will aid you to heal wounds and avoid infections. When the stressor is prolonged, then it will weaken your immunity, and you will be prone to illnesses such as common cold and flu. Now that we have seen what stress can do to your body, we now go-ahead to look at the various mindfulness meditation techniques that are good for stress relief.

The following techniques are ideal for someone that is trying to be familiar with mindful meditation, or it can be useful for those that have practiced mindful meditation before and might not have used the techniques yet.

Let us check out these techniques and how they can work for you.

Chapter 3: The Main Categories of Meditation

Meditation can be approached in lots of ways. There's no one right way of doing it, but there are a few methods that work for most people. Should one type of meditation lose its luster over time, or routine accidentally slip into mindlessness, there are dozens of other ways to meditate that can be familiar to the type you already know or seem totally fresh. All types of meditation are intricately interrelated, but can be sorted generally into five major categories for an easier review.

These five kinds are: spiritual practice, meditation in motion, visualization meditation, verbal meditation, and Awareness meditation.

Meditate for The First Time

For now, we're going to talk about how to meditate for the very first time, even if you've never done it before. This is why you're here, and you'll be happy to hear that it's a LOT easier than you think to get started. You can actually get started right now, wherever you are. Even if you're not at home, there is a way for you to start meditating even while walking around! It's easier to do at home when you're completely relaxed but you don't have to do that. It can be done anywhere just try to avoid doing it while your boss is speaking to you and getting on your nerves! (Yes, this actually happened.)

What to Actually DO (Step by Step)

Find Somewhere Comfortable

You ideally need to find somewhere comfortable to meditate. You'll have much better results if you do this somewhere you feel at home and relaxed, but of course, you can do it anywhere. Try and find somewhere you won't be interrupted, as interruption can be very disrupting for the flow you are trying to create. I've found that if I'm interrupted halfway through meditating, I lose the benefits for that session and can't easily get back into the relaxed state of mind. I have to completely start again, and it takes more time. This can be difficult when you have children but I try to explain to them that I am taking a few minutes for my mental health and that it will benefit them in the long run if they just give me a few minutes! Does it always work? No! But usually they are really good with giving me the time I need.

So, make sure to find somewhere you're not going to be interrupted or interfered with. This can also include things like your phone, noises, lights and other interruptions that might not be obvious now. Put your devices on silent and turn your phone over you the light doesn't interrupt you either. Have a sip or two of water so you're not thirsty during the meditation. It's important to drink enough water during the day by the way! Don't forget.

Find something to sit on, but ideally, a chair or a cushion. The main idea is to get comfortable but not TOO comfortable (unless you are using meditation to sleep) Many people sit on the floor cross legged. I personally use a yoga mat on the floor. I found that if I got too comfy (say in a comfy chair or in my comfy bed) it was easy for my mind to drift into daydreams or my plans for the day etc. I will say that I have gotten much better at this though as time has progressed.

So, try and find something like a cushion, or even sit on the grass outside. I find that being outside is a beautiful place for meditating, just a grassy field or a park or something like that. I enjoy connecting with the earth. You may feel better doing this outside as well, as long as the place you're doing it is peaceful and calm. I love doing it near water as well. There is just something about hearing the waves crash for me, but find what works best for you. .

Find somewhere that you're not going to be distracted or interrupted. The goal when you sit down is to keep your back straight and upright, and your chest out. This lets you breathe deeply and fully, and doesn't restrict you in any way. It also helps you to relax but doesn't let you fall asleep or drift. Also, make sure you do actually breathe deeply but don't force it. Just breathe as deeply as you can comfortably do! If you are uncomfortable, go ahead and sit in a chair just try to remain focused.

Go ahead and set a timer on your phone. If you are like me, your mind will wonder and you will be checking your phone every few minutes to see "are we there yet?" Actually, at the start, the problem you'll have is that you'll try and stop meditating before it's even been 5 minutes. You need a timer to tell you that you're not done yet! Set a soft alarm or tone on your phone to go off after about 10 minutes. You might have to start with a lower time like 5 minutes if you're not used to this, because it can be difficult at first. Like we said about the default mode network, it's called 'default' for a reason. It's the system you most often use, and it's powerful.

So, after a few seconds of doing 'nothing' your brain starts to act up and makes you think about all sorts of things. You'll start freaking out or thinking about all the things you need to do today. So set an alarm for 10 minutes, and tell yourself you're not going to stop meditating until the timer goes off. Be strict with yourself because otherwise, you'll only do it for a few seconds. You need to start flexing that meditation muscle and you do that by setting a timer and sticking to it.

If you're doing this during the day it might actually be difficult to keep your eyes closed (especially if it is a bright and shiny day and you keep thinking about how much you want to go play outside!) If you can't close your eyes, practice looking or gazing at a spot on your wall but not moving your eyes around. Don't look at the details, just let the object fade away so you can't really notice it any more. An easy way of doing this at first is to just stare at a candle flame. A candle flame is amazing in the sense that it has the ability to relax your mind and help you just focus on nothingness. When I first started I did use a candle, but now I am able to just shut my eyes and find that sweet spot. Over time, you'll get used to closing your eyes for long periods of time so you'll be able to do it in the middle of the day in a park for example.

Get Comfortable and Sit Up Straight

Make sure you're comfortable and sitting with your back straight. This is a good time to make sure you're not uncomfortable or slouching. Make sure your back is straight but not forced. It should feel quite nice to straighten your back and hold it straight, but if you're not used to doing that or you have poor posture then this might feel a little unusual.

Focus on Breathing

This is an important step! This is where you start the meditation practice. Focus on your breathing. That's all you need to do is just focus on how your breathing feels. Just be aware of your breathing, and experience how it feels, how it sounds and how it must look for your chest to move in and out while you're breathing. This is where most people fail at meditation, but bear in mind you can't really 'fail'. You can just lose focus for a moment and it's at those moments that you need to bring your focus back to the breathing. All you're going to do is count your breaths from 1 to 10. Count 1 with the 'in breath', then 2 with the 'out breathe' and so on. When you get to 10, start again at 1.

Counting breaths is just a good way of getting beginners to focus on something measurable. It is not necessary however, it definitely helps.

Your mind may wander now, even when you focus on your breathing. This is very normal, and a lot of people, both beginners and advanced meditators, have this problem from time to time. It's easy to lose focus and start thinking about a million other things. But don't beat yourself up about it. It's going to happen. You're going to lose focus, the real growth happens when you notice you're having these thoughts, and then move your attention back to the breathing or whatever visual you are using.

I can't begin to tell you the amount of times I began to think about what I was going to make for dinner, or what the kids will need from me when I was done. I even thought about things from my childhood. As best as you can just bring your attention back to just thinking about your breathing. Focus on staying in the present. Start to focus on how you feel. How relaxed you are. How it sounds when you draw and release your breaths. Again, the key is to stay present. That's the point of meditation, being able to bring that awareness and focus back to one particular thing or point. In this case, that thing is your breathing.

When You Finish.

A really important part of meditation is when the timer goes off. When your timers done and you've done your 10 minutes of meditation ask yourself 'how do I feel?'. Really take note of this. Are you feeling at all refreshed? This helps you stay motivated. The chances are the first few times you'll feel a bit nervous or it might be a little uncomfortable. This is because your brain likely hasn't done this before and it's weird to have experienced a period of ten minutes where you're not thinking about 1000 different things.

Just continue to focus on how you feel. How grateful you are for the things that you have. How grateful your mind feels because you took the time to clear it and give it a break. Call it the law of vibration, karma or the Golden Rule but I believe we always get back what we give out. Being grateful for what you have brings more things in our lives to be grateful for. Practicing gratitude helps me to stay present and mindful. Soon, your brain will come to crave this time and want more of it. My brain actually sends me "Thank You" letters.

What it's going to feel like

A bit strange.
 Meditation is a powerful tool, and if you've never done it, it can clear emotional or mental blocks you've had for years. Some people start crying uncontrollably when they first meditate, because they've never experienced that sense of calm and serenity. It lets you step back and feel your body once more. It lets you step away from the thoughts and monkey mind chatter that's so controlling and manipulative in our lives.

So, you might cry, you might laugh, you might feel good or uncomfortable or you might feel nothing at all. The first time is always the most unpredictable. Whatever your experience of meditation is the first time, just accept it and keep going. It might not be what you expected , it might be better or worse. But the truth is after a while, it will get easier. You will be able to access deeper states of relaxation and serenity. It might take you a few days, weeks or even months, but it will happen as you continue to do it.

If you keep meditating every single morning and evening, you'll definitely feel better. That I can tell you for a fact. I've never met anyone who's meditated every day for more than a month and felt worse. It's always better, always deeper, calmer, and they've always found it easier to focus. Before we go on, make a commitment to trying this for 30 days. Once a day for 30 days and then decide how you feel. I would also advise to keep a journal. Write things down. Journaling is my jam! I write down how I am feeling after my meditation. Be a little bit patient with this and just give yourself a chance to really experience it. It might take longer than you wanted, but stick with it, I promise it gets easier. On the other hand, you might be reading this thinking 'it's fine, I did it with no problems!'. That's great!

Chapter 4: Meditation for Different Ailments

Meditation can be beneficial to various aspects of your life when it is done the right way. Let us look at these benefits so that you know what you are getting into:

Meditation for Anxiety

Anxiety is a condition that won't give you the chance to achieve inner peace at any given time. It is a thief of joy and of time. Let us look at various ways that you can use meditation to achieve the inner peace necessary to avoid anxiety, which can lead to depression. These meditation techniques also help you to avoid panic attacks that might arise. The good thing is most of the meditations help in anxiety, the various exercises differ in their efficacy.

Breathing Meditation for Anxiety

Breathing is one of the most effective meditation techniques. When done the right way, it can assist in calming the anxious mind. It is similar to taking a breath of fresh air once you are anxious. So, when you feel anxious, find ten minutes and just focus on the way you breathe. I recommend the 4-7-8 breathing technique. It involves breathing in for 4 seconds, holding the breath for 7 seconds, and exhaling for 8 seconds. Start slowly making sure to take deep breaths.

Measured Breathing

Here, you have to sit or stand in a comfortable posture. You then have to relax the body. Take a deep breath through the nose while you are counting up to four, feel the air go through to your lungs and let it fill up your stomach. At end of inhalation, grip breath for 3 seconds, and then while still relaxed, let the air slowly out through the nose.

Humming Breath

Very easy, making it a top meditation exercise for beginners as well. It works in the same way as the mindfulness meditation practice, and for you to do the exercise, have 100 percent focus when breathing. While doing this, you need to hum. The process is the same as the breathing exercise, but the only difference is in the humming. Make sure you meditate on the humming, as compared to focusing on the breathing. Do this for several repetitions so that you can feel it.

Diaphragm Breathing

The most common meditation method used to handle anxiety. Follow the same procedure, but when you breathe in, put hand over the stomach so that you can imagine air filling your stomach.

When you exhale, do it through the mouth, with the lips compressed and the jaw relaxed. Redo this several times.

Alternate Nostril Breathing

This is another method that you can use for handling anxiety. In addition to ending the signs of being anxious, it also helps to relieve stress. Do this, close one of the nostrils and then leave the other one open breath by the next nostril. Now change the fingers so that the initial nostril is blocked and use the other one for breathing.
Redo the process.

This is one of the other meditations that you can use to handle the anxiety. You do this by passing the consciousness around your body, a sort of "scan" if you will ,of your body.
When you feel yourself going into a state of anxiety, the key is to use the "scan" to identify it early and address it. It is usually recommended to take 30-40 minutes to do this. Using the body scan, you can be able to identify and handle the early stages of the upcoming attack. When this happens, you can take various steps to handle the anxiety way before it becomes a challenge.

Meditation for Tension Headaches

Tension headache refers to a mild to moderate pain that is in your head. It usually feels as if someone has tied a tight band around the head. The causes of the tension headache aren't so known. The tension headache comes in various forms:

Episodic
These tension headaches can last any time from half an hour to a week. These episodic tension headaches can turn out to be chronic.

Chronic
Chronic tension headaches can last hours on hours. They might be continuous and can occur for more than 15 days each month. Research shows that various types of meditation can help you relieve your tension headaches.

Mindfulness Meditation for Tension Headaches

There are clear associations between headaches and stress. This means that if you reduce your stress, you can relieve the headache. It is also known that those people that suffer from tension headaches aren't able to recover effectively from stressful events. Mindfulness meditation can help you to increase the effectiveness of reducing and healing tension headaches.

Steps to Recovery
When you decide to take up mindfulness meditation for tension headache, you need to know what to do and how to do it. Here are a few steps:

Have a Pain Diary
Before you get right into the process of healing, you need to have a pain diary that will aid you track the intensity of pain, how frequent it occurs, the duration of each headache and any associated symptoms. Some of the associated symptoms include vertigo, nausea, photophobia, and tingling. When you have a pain diary, you get to establish the level of the pain. The usual pain scale for us in the medical field is the 1-10 pain scale. One being that you are barely feeling any pain and ten being that you are in so much pain you can't

do anything or think of anything else. Side note: I once saw a meme of a pain scale that showed 1=being on your cell phone playing candy crush and 10=stigmata and that is what I refer to in my mind now!

Meditate
You need to follow the basic mindfulness meditation techniques that we have outlined in this book. Make sure you earn the techniques and follow them as best you can. Don't get discouraged !

Track
When you start meditating, you need to note down in the diary. Learn to note everything before you start and when you finish.

Analyze
After you get enough data, try and compare the results and see if the tension headaches reduced in any way. Make sure you consider all the aspects that you noted down, including the frequency, the duration, and any other symptoms.

Repeat
Try and repeat the process until you get satisfied with the process.

Meditation for Reducing Tension

Headaches are as a result of bodily tension that comes when you clench your muscles. This is usually seen when the tension is in the neck, jaw, and face. Using meditation, you can relax the whole body. When you get into the meditation process, you naturally release anything that causes the headache. When you reduce the chances of tension in your body, you also reduce the possibility of having a headache. You also get a chance to stop the headache fast.

Meditation for Better Sleep

Sleep is one of the ways to make you healthy and fit. When you rest well, you have the capacity to have a good day ahead of you. Waking up when you are fresh is the first step to a good day.
Let us look at the various meditation techniques that will aid you enjoy better sleep.

Meditation for Better Sleep
Guided meditation for sleep is a way to help you let go of any worrying thoughts and relax the body before you can sleep. Just like other forms of meditation that you have come across, you need to move the focus from the mind to the sensations in the body. When you practice this meditation regularly, you tend to sleep better.

Research by the American Sleep Association shows that more than 30 percent of the adults have problems with falling asleep or maintaining sleep. Research also shows that more than 30 percent of the adults will get less than 7 hours of sleep each night.

When you sleep better, you will be able to improve your immunity, and you will function at your best. If you have a problem with anxiety, you will be able to handle it better if you meditate before you sleep.

The aim of guided sleep meditation is to reduce the effect of worries and tension that build up in your body before you can sleep. When you learn to focus and then relax the body, you will notice massive improvements in the ability to sleep.

The Benefits

Guided meditation for sleep allows you to move out of the past and the future and focus on the present. Usually, when you lie down to sleep, you may swim in thoughts that were suppressed in the daytime. "Did I document in that patients chart correctly?" "Wonder which one of the kids has homework they didn't tell me about that is due tomorrow" Without any help, controlling these thoughts can be hard.

When you use guided sleep meditation, you get to let go of the thoughts that are going through your head. When you relax, the heart rate goes down, and the breathing rate also slows. All of these make you ready to sleep better.

Many of the guided sleep meditation exercises will have you follow an audio guide that you can use on the radio or through your phone. You get guided via the voice in the audio. A good tip here is to choose one with a nice ASMR voice…something I failed to do when I first started ! I made myself a note to DM Idris Elba on instagram to see if he would be willing to upload one to YouTube for our listening pleasure.

The Process

You need to lie down comfortably and play the audio. This way, you get to redirect the attention away from your thoughts to your body using what is called a body scan. This process means you let go of your thoughts and then focus on the sensations in the body without the need to change them. Try and move through the different parts of the body, starting from the head to the toes. Make sure you notice the different sensations that you feel when moving through the feelings. The audio will tell you which part to go through and what sensations to look out for. Apart from the body scan, you can use the breathing exercise, visualization, and gratitude as some form of meditation.

Meditation for Mental Aspect of Life

When you relax and focus on your inner peace, you can improve your mental health. In research that was later published in the JAMA Internal Medicine in 2014, researchers found that meditation programs helped reduce the symptoms of anxiety and depression. Another scientific study published in 2018 in the Psychiatric Review, found out that subjects that suffered from generalized anxiety enjoyed a better reduction in stressful symptoms. Let us look at the various ways that meditation can help in handling mental issues.

Meditation and Negative Emotions

Meditation has the capability to handle negative emotions in a way that is healthy and effective. You need to remember that emotions are the core of your actions. Your whole human experience is enshrined in emotions, right from your childhood. You have experienced waves of happiness, sadness, anger, and more.

When you meditate, you learn how to identify emotions deep within yourself so that you can study them, learn more about them, and then release them. The various ancient traditions of the east, such as Daoism, Buddhism, and Hinduism, have long studied man's emotions, and they do this with the aim of going past human suffering.

The Techniques include

Seeing Clearly

Here, you have to look at the emotion in a different way. First, you have to recognize the emotion that you have encountered, then label the emotion before you can go ahead to handle it. The negative emotion can be fear, sadness, or anything else. Before you can handle it, go ahead and identify it and when you do you will handle it much easier. When you label the emotion, don't own it; instead, use words that will make the emotion look easier to handle.

After you label the emotion, the next thing is you have to take a few breaths and then divert your attention from the emotion. This means you don't pay any attention to the root cause of the emotion; rather, you need to look at the attention itself. You accept that the feeling is there, but you don't put your emotion on it.

Examine

After you put a name to the emotion, the next thing is to try and know what caused it. Look at the issues that trigger the feeling at any moment, and then note them down if possible.. Once you look at the various causes of the emotion, try and identify them, and handle them. The next thing is to try and look at what the effects of the emotions are in your body. What do you feel when the emotion happens? Where does the feeling take you, and how does it feel? What do you think about the feeling?

Next, look deep into yourself and understand what the feeling is all about. Can you put a size to the feeling? The color and consistency? If the emotion wasn't there at the moment, where did it come from? Learn as much as you can about the emotion. Remember that emotions make the bulk of our lives and you need to know so much about it so that you aren't a slave to it.

Release

Ah, release. If only this were easy right? First, you will be clear with the emotion; you will be composed when you have the emotion in check, and you know what it is. You also get to know the emotion what triggers it and the effects it has on your life. The final stage is to liberate yourself from the emotion.

Many times, you can find out that the emotion points to something which needs attention from you in your life. This will prompt you to take action. There are many ways to take action here. Channeling that energy into a creative process (writing, music, art etc.) is one way. Therapy with a trusted professional is another. I cannot stress enough how important it is to have someone you trust and who you feel will really take the time to work through these things with you. TRUST IS A MUST!!

Acknowledge the Temporary Nature of the Emotion
When you have a negative emotion burdening you, the next thing is that you need to know that the emotions which you experience are not permanent. The negative emotions will come up, be around for a while then disappear. They are like waves of the sea they come and go. Your role in this sense is just to be a witness to the wave of the emotion. You observe it as it changes its form and washes through you. When you use mindfulness, you will be able to view the emotion as a series of mental events that pass through in a temporary manner.

Trust Yourself
When you have the emotion in check, the next step would be to trust your own self. The aim is to identify the emotion then come up with various solutions that can allow you to handle the issue. These solutions need to be ideal for your situation.

Guided Imagery for Handling Mental Issues
This meditation method makes use of a pleasing scene or image to help you focus on that instead of what might be happening mentally. When you get to the practitioner, he takes your history so that he can get to know what the issue at hand is. When you talk to the therapist about your issue, he comes up with a series of images that you can follow.

As an example, the therapist will ask you to picture a serene day in a garden on a sunny day. You have to describe the sounds, sights, and aromas that arouse from the scenery. The therapist will try to invoke a few sensory aspects of the environment. You might also ask for some music to accompany the scenery being played out in your mind. The aim is to engage all your five senses. The therapist observes you to signs of emotion, which will be reflected in the way you change your body position. He also notes the change in voice and the breathing. With time, your breath slows down, and the muscles loosen while the mental activity reduces. Guided meditation is ideal for both groups as well as a personal meditation.

Uses
Guided meditation is ideal for treating grief, anxiety, depression, addiction, and many other stress disorders. It can also help someone to stop smoking as well as reduce the awareness of pain.

Progressive Muscle Relaxation

This type of meditation uses the aspect of tensing different muscle groups, holding the contraction for a few seconds then releasing it while you exhale. The therapist notes the things that happen when you do it. After a short while, the therapist will focus on another muscle group. He repeats the process in a systematic manner, starting from the toes upwards. You tighten the muscle gently so that you don't end up with the strain. The therapist will note the difference between the relaxation and the tautness. At the end of everything, the client will feel body-wide tranquility.

Uses

You can use the relaxation technique to know what happens when the muscles are under tension or relaxed. Tightening and releasing the strain will help handle negative emotions such as anger, anxiety, and frustration.

As an example, if you usually clench your fists after an altercation, you can use this meditation method to prevent this and release the agitation.

Additionally, you can use the meditation method to relieve social anxiety, panic attacks, and insomnia.

Hypnosis

The method is a little similar to guided meditation, but in this case, you use verbal cues as opposed to visual stimulation. This method is ideal for people that need to change their behavior, adopt new habits, and to relieve symptoms. The first step is the therapist to put you into a state of deep relaxation. After you slip into the trance, you will get goal-oriented suggestions that you need to follow.

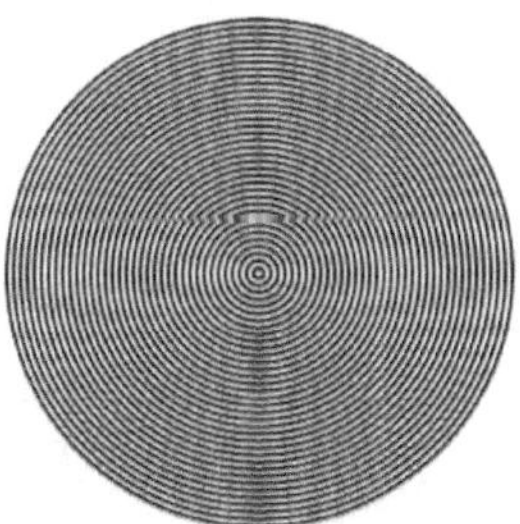

The hypnosis might take the whole session or a few minutes of the session. When you get used to hypnosis, you will learn to do it by yourself. Many therapists will have audio files that include instructions.

Uses

The meditation technique can help you beat stress, addiction, and phobias as well as anxiety. It can also help you quit smoking.

Mindfulness

This technique allows you to watch your thoughts, sensations as well as emotions without having to attach to them. It is the awareness of some-thing.

It is deliberately paying attention to your thoughts and sensations without passing judgment on them. Some of the mental anchors that you can use include a vase or a ticking clock. When you get to the point of watching your thoughts, you get the ability to change your behavior and beliefs.

Uses
Therapists can use the method to handle depression, anxiety, panic attacks, addiction, and many more.

Focused Breathing
This form of breathing is also referred to as paced breathing. When you undertake focused breathing, you will do it in a slow, gentle, and smooth manner.
You can do this on your own or in a group, supervised by a therapist. When you inhale, the therapist looks at the body for areas of tension such as the lips, jaws, and shoulders. When you exhale, you release the tightness in the various body parts, which in turn helps you to focus on the sensation. You can make the meditation better by using one nostril at a time. Close one of the nostrils and then breathe through the open one, then do the opposite. Make sure you inhale and exhale so that you feel all the sensations.

Uses
You can apply the meditation technique to build alertness and decrease negative thoughts. You can use the meditation method to handle panic attacks, anxiety, and addiction.

Meditation for Depression

It is beneficial to use meditation in conjunction with anti-depressant medication. Please keep in mind that using meditation will not replace any medications for depression that you have been advised to use. Meditation has been in use for many years to reduce the symptoms of depression, but it shouldn't replace conventional medication. Let us look at the various aspects of meditation that can be ideal for treating depression.

Loving-kindness Meditation
This form of meditation will create a sense of love and kindness towards yourself and other people around you. The expected results include a more positive outlook on life, better compassion, and fewer negative emotions. Learning to love yourself and honor yourself is one of THE best things you can do for yourself and those around you. You can combine this with compassion meditation, which teaches you to have unconditional compassion for yourself and really focuses on giving yourself grace. I am a big fan of something called "mirror work" where you look in a mirror and speak to yourself in a loving manner. I found this very difficult at first, but am quite the pro at it now as I speak to myself as I would speak to one of my children or someone that I love dearly.

Mindfulness

Mindfulness keeps you present. It allows you to have an awareness of the moment. A few minutes each day will aid you to train your mind. Inhale and exhale as you feel the various sensations run through your body. Open up and accept your emotions while not passing judgment on them or attaching to them. This has various benefits that include lower emotional reaction. You don't have to set aside a specific time of day or place to be aware of the breathing throughout the day. You can do this while sitting, standing, or lying down.

The Spiritual Meditation Technique

In my research I have come across those who practice this. They say this brings you to your "real self", the depths of who you really are. It comes from the innate longing to see, feel and think something beyond this physical realm.

Here are the steps to successful spiritual meditation

Get a Quiet Place

Find a place that is comfortable for you. Make sure you avoid places that are noisy or that have a lot of distractions. Get in your comfortable position. This is not a meditation that I would do while sitting up or standing. This is one that I get really comfortable with. Like in bed comfortable! This really puts the focus on your inner being and for some reason it makes me really sleepy so I usually do this at night before bed or if I am doing during the day I make sure I don't have any prior commitments. Once you are seated comfortably, you can close your eyes and start experiencing the emotions.

Experience the Process

Now that you have found the right position to help you meditate, the next thing is to let go. Loosen up and then let everything take a natural course. I am not here to force my belief system on anyone but I personally ask God to "Come sit with me and show me what I need to see" You need to be a passive spectator, allowing the process to go ahead on its own. Don't be concerned about what will happen or getting things right let it follow its natural course.

Acknowledge Your Thoughts

The aim of meditation is to leave the thoughts to go away; let the ideas get into your thought process, but take time to control the urge to react to the various thoughts. We are so bombarded with information from our televisions, cell phones and even other people. Try not to let the thoughts consume and control you. Acknowledge them and focus on the meditation.

Utter a Prayer

As you are preventing your thoughts from taking over, say something that will mean something to you. The prayer can be a phrase or a single word. It doesn't necessarily have to do with a religious affiliation. I once worked with a patient with severe PTSD who would repeat the date and year as it was comforting to her to reassure herself that her abusive past was behind her. It can be a mantra or even a word or phrase that brings you comfort in some way. When you do this, make sure your body remains relaxed and loose, and breathe naturally and slowly.

Reflect on Your Progress
Look at yourself after the whole process. Find out how the body feels and be attentive to the breath and thoughts. Stay calm and relax, and then open your eyes and let the effects of meditation sink in. Feel how you become less agitated after the session.

Chapter 5: Common Problems People Have in Meditation

Mind is Racing

Many people, when they first try the technique just described, report their mind was racing. They were unable to think about just one thing, and instead they focused on everything. Their body and how it felt, their phone, thoughts about what to have for dinner or what to do tomorrow. Everything. That's really common, and for a lot of people it's just a prime example of how the default mode network operates. It's designed to get you to think about various different things and constantly get distracted. It's attracted to novelty and distracting things like TV shows and instant gratification.

There's not really an easy fix for this, my advice is to power through and build the muscle slowly. I would recommend trying some guided meditation to begin with. There are some good ones on YouTube. Think of meditating like a physical muscle, you can't lift a heavy weight on day one, can you? So, don't try and meditate perfectly the first time. Just focus on doing one thing: Every time you notice yourself thinking about something else, try and gently move your focus back to your breathing. After a while of doing this, (this is why you should try for at least a month) it gets easier. Suddenly you don't think about that other stuff as often, and when you do, it's easier to move your focus back to your breathing.

Falling Asleep

A really common problem people have when they try and meditate first thing in the morning is, they fall back asleep! If you also get up early, it's super easy to just go back to sleep if you're all warm and comfortable in your chair or laying in your bed. But that's why it's important to not sit in a chair or lay on a bed, unless you are using meditation to sleep. If you're having trouble staying awake while doing this, you need to sit on a cushion on the floor, with your back straight.

 One thing I have learned is that meditation is not sleeping, it's quite the opposite. It's the act of deciding to sit there, awake, thinking about no-thing. That being said, I personally use meditation at night when I am ready to fall asleep. I had quite a serious issue with insomnia and this has helped. For this reason, I meditate twice daily. Once in the morning, before I start my day and then again at night to get me relaxed enough to sleep. Again, find what works for you!

Can't Sit Down for Long Enough

Probably one of the most common problems you'll find is that you just can't sit down for long enough. This is another thing that can only really be fixed with practice and determination. Tell yourself that you've got to stick to it for at least a month. After this time, you'll find it much easier, and you'll be able to sit still for long periods of time.

It Hurts My Knees or Back

If you're in pain, you should stop. Try taking it slowly, and making sure that when you set yourself up for meditation, you're not sitting in a way that might get uncomfortable after a few minutes. This takes a bit of practice to get to the point where you can tell what's going to be uncomfortable before doing it. You want to get to the point where you can sort of 'sense' what position is going to be uncomfortable, before getting into it. The best position is just the cross-legged sitting position on a cushion or something like that, with a straight back and your chest out.

For 90% of people, there will be literally no problems with this position. But for some people, maybe people with back pain or posture issues, this might be a problem. Just take it at your own pace and find what works for you. It's going to be different for everyone. If it hurts your knees, because sitting cross legged is hard for you, then find something to sit on that is comfortable for you. I do encourage you to sit up if you are not planning to use this for sleep though. By sitting with your back straight and with nothing supporting your back, you force yourself to be aware of what you're doing and think about what you're doing. This makes it easier to stay present and mindful of what it is that you are trying to accomplish here.

I Don't Have Time

Ah, time. The classic default excuse for almost everything. I don't have time. It's been said that if you don't have time to meditate, you need it more than anyone else. Everyone has time to meditate, and if you don't, you can make time. It only takes a few minutes a day and if you're saying 'I don't even have 5 spare minutes in my day' then just get up 5 minutes earlier.

Listen I understand the time thing. It's hard to work full time plus be a full time parent, but we can ALL squeeze in a few minutes at some point in our day! Try it when you first get up before you even check your phone. This is when I find it has the biggest effect. It sets me up for the day and makes everything else easier. But it's also been said that meditation GIVES you more time than it takes away. This is because it makes you more alert and aware during the other things you're doing with your day. Therefore, if you don't think you have time, think again!

Nothing's Happening

You've been sitting there for ten minutes, your timers gone off but nothing's happened. What's wrong? Are you doing it wrong? You start to question why you bothered buying this book or even thinking about learning how to meditate. Don't worry, this happens a lot. I recall sitting there after my first time and thinking, "Ok is that it or what?" That's why it's important to keep doing it. Commit to it. You can't expect the mind that has been in chaos and conflict for years (47 in my case!) will suddenly shift itself into finding peace after 10 minutes, but wouldn't that be nice?!

So those are the most common problems people have. If you've had one or more of those problems when trying to meditate, please keep going. Don't focus on it. Most of the problems you'll have will be the mental ones. Things like not being able to sit still long enough or not being able to concentrate on what you're doing. Those only get easier with time and practice, so just keep going with them!

How to Practice This Every Day?

This Needs to Be Practiced Literally Every Single Day.

Of course, you can miss a day here and there, but the main benefits are mainly felt when you practice this every day for about 60 days or so. There are a few ways of doing that. You need to firstly set yourself a challenge to meditate every day for 60 days. You can write a chart or tick off days on a calendar that you've meditated, if that makes it easier. I used just a regular old calendar. I marked an "X" on the dates I meditated when I first started. It was psychological. I'm telling you this mind of mine...........!!! Now I meditate daily so there is no need to mark a calendar.

Once the habit is built, it's very hard to not meditate. I feel very strange and uncomfortable if I don't meditate in the morning now. My brain gets super pissed at me when I miss my meditation time. It really sets me up for the day and helps me to focus on what I am doing so when I DON'T do it, I really feel discombobulated and end up setting aside at least a few minutes to get it done. Here's something to remember: Meditating once per day for 3 minutes is going to be more beneficial to you than meditating once a week for an hour. This really needs to be a daily thing. If you can only commit to doing about 3 minutes a day, that's fine but make sure it literally is every single day. Ideally, you want to be meditating for about 20-30 minutes a day every day. This can be spread out into 15 minutes in the morning and 15 in the evening. Or, you could even meditate for 10 minutes in the morning, 10 before lunch and 10 before bed.

However, you break it up, the key is to get a certain number of minutes per day not per week. It really only changes the brain if you do it every day, and it's not something like emails that you can just bunch up to the end of the week, and reply to them all then. You can't 'binge meditate' at the weekend! Your brain is not Netflix!!

There's not really a secret for how to do this every day. You've just got to set the target and do it. After all, it's you that has everything to gain here, so just ask yourself 'Do I want to feel better?'.But even on days when you don't really feel like it, it's important to do it then too. When you don't feel like meditating, that's probably a good sign that you really need to make time to do it. If you're having a really bad day and you just don't want to meditate, that's when it's needed the most. It will most certainly make you feel better! From now on, make the commitment to giving your brain the break it so desperately needs and deserves. .You've already learned all you need to know about meditation, and it's now just up to you to actually practice it every single day.

Conclusion

When you hear the word meditation, you think of monks who are in flowing robes hidden away from civilization sitting pensively without a sound. They seem at peace and far removed from normal life. That is just one single aspect of meditation. Meditation refers to the act of bringing your attention to one simple focus. Some use candles. Some use words. Some focus on feelings or breathing. The end result is this: meditation practice is all about focusing your mind. It is about letting go of the chaos of uncontrolled thoughts. You may still have thoughts upon thoughts, but you will just acknowledge that they exist, and then let them go and bring your focus back to the present. The aim is to create a "pause" in your thinking, to slow down the pace of thought so that we can sink in and relax, rest and re-balance.

In short, meditation has the power to not only better YOUR life, it also has the potential to better the people that are around you. I am sure you have heard the saying ," If mama ain't happy, nobody is happy." It is true. I can promise you that if you ask any one of my children if they would prefer the mother that I am now compared to the mother that I was prior to meditating, the answer would be a resounding "YES" Not only am I a better mother but I am also a better friend and person in general, and for that I will ever be grateful.